PPINESS

14 LESSONS
— IN —
HAPPINESS

A GUIDEBOOK ON IMPROVING YOUR LIFE

GINA ROSS

Copyright © 2022 by Gina Ross

All rights reserved. No part of this book may be reproduced or used in any manner without written permission of the copyright owner except for the use of quotations in a book review. For more information, address:
wd3hypnotherapy@gmail.com

FIRST EDITION

Paperback ISBN: 978-1-80227-488-2
eBook ISBN: 978-1-80227-489-9

www.rickmansworthhypnotherapy.co.uk

*I dedicate this book of lessons to my children,
the greatest teachers in happiness
I have ever had.*

Disclaimer

Any use of information in this book is at the readers discretion and risk and the author is exempt from any responsibility of actions taken by the reader in conjunction with this work.

This book is simply intended to motivate and guide my readers.

It is not designed to give any type of psychological, legal or medical advice.

Nothing written within this book is intended to be used as a cure for depression, anxiety or any mental illness whatsoever.

Accordingly, please use it as a supplement and not as a substitute for any professional psychological, legal or medical advice.

Always consult a professional practitioner.

The content of each lesson is the opinion and expression of the author and is considered fair, true and accurate. The author can not be held responsible nor gives any warranties or guarantees expressed or implied by the author's choice to include any content from any material on third party websites or from any other source whatsoever.

Neither the author or publisher shall be liable for any physical, psychological, emotional, financial or commercial damages, including, but not limited to, special, incidental, consequential or other damages.

Table of Contents

PREFACE — ix

INTRODUCTION — 1

LESSON ONE: Reframe Your Thoughts — 7

LESSON TWO: Pay Attention to Your Breathing — 11

LESSON THREE: Practise Meditation — 17

LESSON FOUR: Be Mindful — 27

LESSON FIVE: Cultivate Self-Love — 35

LESSON SIX: Be More Confident — 49

LESSON SEVEN: Pursue Your Dreams — 63

LESSON EIGHT: Be Kind — 73

Lesson Nine: Learn to Deal with Negative Emotions   83

Lesson Ten: Learn to Deal with Other People's Negativity   95

Lesson Eleven: Practise Forgiveness   109

Lesson Twelve: Conquer Fear and Anxiety   115

Lesson Thirteen: Embrace Failure   123

Lesson Fourteen: Accept Death   129

Final Thoughts   143

Preface

"Happiness begins with you. Not with your relationship, your friends or your job, but with you"

—Mandy Hale

My overarching aim in writing this book is to highlight to you, the reader, that you alone are responsible for your own happiness.

Irrespective of any negativity and challenges that you have already experienced or will experience on your journey through life, it is within your own power to feel happy or sad, depending on your thoughts.

Despite the simplicity and logic of the above idea, it has actually taken me, a former sufferer of crippling anxiety, years of attending courses and reading countless books to fully understand it and to become enlightened, in a sense.

This enlightenment has led me to write this book, with simple tips and a multitude of practical exercises designed to enable you to improve your mindset and overcome any difficulties as they arise.

The exercises throughout this book have all been tried and tested on both myself and on many of my hypnotherapy clients, so I can also confirm that they actually work.

That being said, the exercises within this book are in no way a substitute for professional medical advice.

Hence, should you be suffering from any mental illness whatsoever, I implore you to contact a medical professional in the first instance.

The idea of writing a guidebook on being happier initially arose as a result of several conversations I had with my clients. Anxiety reduction, increased confidence and self-esteem (to name a few of their goals) often seemed to be a smokescreen for their ultimate goal to be happy.

Preface

As a former teacher, I have arranged the contents of this book in the form of a series of 14 lessons.

The lessons can be worked through in their sequential order, or you can simply choose to work through the specific lessons that are relevant to you.

By committing to practising the exercises and by following the tips and advice laid out herein, you may find that you experience one or more of the following benefits:

1. An increase in inner calm.
2. An ability to reduce anxiety.
3. Strength to conquer fears and phobias.
4. An improvement in your relationships.
5. An overall unleashing of self-love and self-confidence.

Overall, the lessons will teach you how to be your most authentic and happiest self, enabling you to reach and live out your ultimate dreams.

Introduction

"Happiness is not out there for us to find. The reason that it's not out there is that it's inside us."

—SONJA LYUBOMIRSKY

Happiness expert, Sonja Lyubomirsky, a professor of psychology at the University of California-Riverside, concluded that even though we all have a happiness set point (a default level of happiness set by our genes), this genetic predisposition only accounts for around 50% of the amount of happiness we can experience and hence, this default level can be improved.

According to the study carried out by Sonja Lyubomirsky,[1] life circumstances and leisure activities

---

1 *Pursuing Happiness: The Architecture of Sustainable Change.* Sonja Lyubomirsky, Kennon M. Sheldon, David Schkade.

account for the remaining 50% of happiness available to us and accordingly, the study suggests that there is also a mental aspect to happiness, a choice.

We all have the capacity to be happier by deliberately choosing to be.

I, myself, grew up expecting happiness to happen naturally and effortlessly.

As a very young child, I was frequently happy.

I recall laughing until my stomach ached. I remember getting the giggles, always seemingly at the worst possible times, times when we were supposed to be quiet and serious.

As a child, I was lighthearted, always managing to see the funny side of things.

Growing older, laughter became a much less frequent event, usually replaced with sober thoughts and occasional tears.

As a teenager and an adult, my earlier playfulness had been replaced with overthinking, and my childhood curiosity and adventurousness replaced with fearfulness.

I didn't understand what had changed.

Genetically, it was probably predetermined that I would naturally be more pessimistic. After all, I was born into a family who always seemed to view the glass as half empty.

They were always on alert, afraid to be truly happy and carefree, as if a tragedy would befall them a second later.

Growing up, I was continually bombarded with negative news, from the constant murmurs of upcoming marriage break-ups to the stream of those diagnosed with one horrific illness after another.

And, if that wasn't enough, my parents' newspaper of choice, The Daily Mail, was filled, end to end, with stories on murderers and corrupt World Leaders.

We seemed to be frequently on the brink of war or on the precipice of some other disaster.

I felt safer embracing negativity, hiding my happiness and suppressing my enthusiasm, just in case something went wrong.

I didn't realise the impact of my negativity until it culminated in my first full-blown panic attack in 2001.

It was at the end of a Summer spent travelling around Egypt, and, on this particular night, I was resting at the top of a mountain, having just spent hours with a group of tourists, climbing to the top.

The sun was just setting, and the low level of oxygen at the top of the mountain, together with the negativity that had been mounting up throughout my life, came to a head, and I had a most intense panic attack.

I recall being led to a Bedouin's tent, where an Egyptian doctor rubbed my back as I rocked back and forth in terror, choking on lemon tea.

I was so unhappy. I was struggling to breathe and my mind was completely riddled with fearful thoughts.

I truly believed that this was it. I was going to die.

Introduction

I prayed to the God who I wasn't even sure I believed in and promised him that if a miracle occurred and I somehow managed to survive, I would work to become a happier person and make the most of every second of my life.

Luckily, both the Bedouin and the Egyptian doctor seemed to be familiar with panic attacks. They were incredibly kind and did everything they could to comfort me, and, as a result, a few hours later, the fear and sadness dissipated.

The rest of the holiday remained fairly calm.

The panic and unhappiness had gone away into an abyss, where they remained for the next ten years.

However, they were not to remain there permanently.

A little over a decade later, the panic returned with a vengeance.

For three months, I was in a state of constant alert, continuously paralysed by fear. I was barely able to eat, unable to relax and suffering from extreme insomnia.

Determined to beat it once and for all and to live happily, I attended various courses and read as many books as I could find on the subject.

It was as a by-product of my search to be happier that I learned that it was actually within my own power to be happy. I learned that happiness is innate and that it is a choice.

And from that point onwards, I made the choice to be happier.

Lesson One

Reframe Your Thoughts

"Very little is needed to make a happy life; it is all within yourself in your way of thinking."

—Marcus Aurelius

Marcus Aurelius was a Roman Emperor and a Stoic Philosopher during the 2nd century AD.

The principles of Stoicism dictate that we all have the capacity to overcome feelings of unhappiness and subsequent suffering, simply by focusing on those things within our control, such as our thoughts, words and actions, and by letting go of those things that we are unable to control, such as the thoughts, words and actions of others.

Stoics believe that simply by reframing thoughts in a more positive direction, we can change our moods, our relationships with others, our overall view of the world and our entire life.

In our day-to-day lives, where there is so little under our control, the idea of being able to control our thoughts and subsequent actions, resulting in an uplift in our feelings, takes on an even greater significance.

To see how your current stream of thoughts is affecting your feelings at this exact moment in time, try the following exercise:

LESSON ONE: REFRAME YOUR THOUGHTS

> *Thought Awareness Exercise*
>
> 1. *Write down your current stream of thoughts.*
> 2. *Write down a few words to describe your current mood and your emotions.*
> 3. *Read back what you have written.*
> 4. *You will notice that your thoughts and your mood correlate.*
>
>   *Hence, if you are thinking negative thoughts, you are likely to be feeling unhappy. Whereas, if you are thinking positive thoughts, you are likely to be feeling happy and empowered.*

In your day-to-day life, notice how often you label a person or an experience as negative and then react emotionally to match that belief.

The following exercise will teach you how to release negativity by replacing negative thoughts with more empowering alternatives.

Reframing Exercise

1. *Split a piece of paper into two columns.*

2. *On one side, write every negative thought you have throughout the day.*

3. *On the other side, write a positive or neutral alternative.*

4. *You will notice that your thoughts are repetitive and that by changing them to more empowering alternatives, your mind will become accustomed to looking at things more optimistically, and your mood and your emotions will begin to improve accordingly.*

Lesson Two

Pay Attention to Your Breathing

"Improper breathing is a common cause of ill health. If I had to limit my advice on healthier living to just one tip, it would be simply to learn how to breathe correctly. There is no single more powerful or more simple daily practice to further your health and well being than breathwork."

—Dr Andrew Weil

Breathing is the most important life skill that we will ever learn.

From the instant we are born, we teach ourselves how to breathe and we continue breathing throughout our lifetime.

Breathing is essential to life.

Every cell in our body relies on oxygen.

Breathing has the power to relieve pain, to provide greater mental focus, to improve sleep and digestion, to increase energy, to lower blood pressure and to reduce stress levels.

In summary, breathing effectively improves and extends our lives.

Dogs, cats and mice breathe rapidly and live a markedly shorter period of time as a result. On average, they only live around 10 years. In comparison, a giant tortoise (that only takes about four to five breaths per minute) can live up to 200 years.

Many of us do not breathe correctly and suffer un-

Lesson Two: Pay Attention to Your Breathing

necessarily as a result. Our breathing is often too fast, resulting in anxiety, depression or both.

By changing our breathing, by slowing it down, we can actually change our moods and improve our life.

In March 2010, sadness and panic struck me for the second time. I had lost my job, my first marriage had failed and my grandmother at 93, who had been such an integral part of our family, had passed away.

My financial situation was so dire that I had to rent my home, after taking a huge remortgage on it, and I moved back in with my parents.

As much as I love my parents and was grateful that they took me back in, I felt unhappy and alone. The sadness would peak at night and I would lie awake, thinking incessantly, seeking to understand what went wrong.

My breathing was both excessive and erratic and I would rock backwards and forwards in fear.

My mouth would feel dry, my body would feel numb and I genuinely thought I was going to die.

I didn't realise that my rapid thoughts, leading to my rapid breathing, were actually creating the anxiety.

It wasn't until around 3 months later, when I was introduced to mindfulness in the form of *Full Catastrophe Living* by Jon Kabat-Zinn, that I realised the profound effect of breathing effectively.

I realised that simply by slowing down my breathing, reducing the length of my inhalations and increasing the length of my exhalations, the fear would dissipate and I would begin to feel better.

According to Jon Kabat-Zinn, correct breathing entails *"intentionally relaxing the belly as much as you can"*. He advises his readers to practise breathing whilst lying down, paying attention to their hands resting on their stomachs as they gently rise upon inhalation and fall upon exhalation.

The following exercise will give you practice in breathing more efficiently, leading to greater peace and relaxation in your day-to-day life.

Lesson Two: Pay Attention to Your Breathing

A Simple Breathing Exercise

1. *Place one hand on your chest and one on your stomach.*

2. *Imagine that there is a balloon in your stomach.*

3. *Breathe into the balloon.*

4. *Imagine the balloon inflating upon inhalation and deflating upon exhalation.*

5. *Breathe into the balloon for the count of 5.*

6. *Hold your breath in for the count of 5.*

7. *Exhale for the count of 7.*

8. *Hold your breath out for the count of 7.*

9. *Repeat the cycle for 5 minutes.*

Lesson Three

Practise Meditation

"The more regularly and the more deeply you meditate, the sooner you will find yourself acting always from a centre of peace."

—J. Donald Walters

Meditating is an essential exercise in calming your mind and your body. A multitude of scientific studies have shown that meditating regularly benefits your body against a range of physical and mental health conditions, including chronic physical pain,[2] anxiety,[3] depression[4] and post-traumatic stress disorder.[5]

Over the years, my anxiety has reared its head again and again.

After my second episode in 2010, it reemerged around two weeks after the birth of my eldest daughter in 2012. The change in hormones post-pregnancy together with all of the sudden commitments and responsibilities of being a first-time mum, again caused an influx of panicked thoughts, followed by a return of the rapid breathing and the symptoms of anxiety that I had experienced before.

This time, rather than simply practising breathing exercises on a sporadic basis, I began to practise them daily.

---

2 https://pubmed.ncbi.nlm.nih.gov/26417764/
3 https://pubmed.ncbi.nlm.nih.gov/24107199/
4 https://pubmed.ncbi.nlm.nih.gov/24395196/
5 https://pubmed.ncbi.nlm.nih.gov/27537781/

Lesson Three: Practise Meditation

As a result, I found that I began to experience an underlying calm in my day-to-day life, and any time I felt the anxiety creeping in, I managed to ward it off more easily.

Since this time, I have resolved to meditate daily. I rise at 6 am and spend 20 minutes concentrating on the word *"calm"*, whilst simply noticing my breathing.

Meditating in the mornings seems to slow down my days which, as a result, tend to be more peaceful.

The following series of meditations will do the same for you. They will calm your mind, giving you peace, clarity and greater focus in everything you do.

An Early Morning Meditation

1. *Begin by closing your eyes and relaxing your whole body.*

2. *Inhale slowly and gently release any tension as you exhale.*

3. *Visualise the smile of someone you love and feel a tingling sensation of happiness within your chest.*

4. *Feel this tingling sensation of happiness behind your eyes and notice as the feeling spreads throughout your whole body.*

5. *Feel the tingling sensation of happiness spread over your entire face.*

6. *Raise the corners of your lips in a smile and feel your eyes soften.*

7. *Rest your tongue behind your teeth and relax your jaw.*

8. *Smile into your throat and voice box. Thank your voice for giving you the ability to speak.*

Lesson Three: Practise Meditation

9. *Feel the tingling sensation of happiness spread to your heart. Feel your heart soften and fill with love. Thank it for keeping you healthy. Upon exhalation, release anger, frustration and pain from your heart.*

10. *Feel the tingling sensation of happiness spreading from your heart to your lungs. Imagine your lungs relaxing. Thank them for allowing oxygen to flow effortlessly through your body.*

11. *Send the tingling sensation of happiness to your liver. Thank your liver for keeping your body healthy.*

12. *Send the tingling sensation of happiness to your stomach and its surrounding organs. Visualise them relaxing and thank them for keeping your body healthy.*

13. *Send the tingling sensation of happiness to your kidneys. Thank them for their role in keeping your body healthy.*

14. *Send the tingling sensation of happiness up your spine, through your bones, muscles, skin and hair.*

15. *Imagine happiness flowing through your whole body.*

16. *Finally, run through the day, visualising how well it is going to go.*

Another Simple Meditation for Greater Peacefulness

1. *Count your breaths (each inhalation and exhalation is one count).*

2. *Count your breaths from 1 to 10.*

3. *Then count your breaths backwards from 10 to 1.*

4. *Repeat 10 times.*

LESSON THREE: PRACTISE MEDITATION

A Meditation to Bring You Energy and Positivity

1. *Inhale, filling an imaginary balloon in your stomach and then exhale.*

2. *Take 10 breaths.*

3. *Imagine inhaling energy and positivity, and releasing tension with every exhalation.*

4. *Allow sounds and voices to remain in the background.*

5. *Invite your toes to relax.*

6. *Invite your feet and your ankles to relax.*

7. *Invite the muscles in your legs to relax.*

8. *Invite your upper legs and knees to relax.*

9. *Invite your hips and pelvis to relax.*

10. *Invite your stomach, back, spine, rib cage, chest, shoulders, neck and arms to relax.*

11. *Invite your hands and fingers to relax.*

12. *Invite your scalp, forehead and face to soften.*

13. Invite your mouth, jaw and teeth to relax.

14. Imagine being in a peaceful place. Imagine that it is a place which is special to you, where you can relax and feel safe.

15. Imagine the colours and shapes in this place.

16. Smell the aroma, feel the temperature and experience comfort from just being there.

17. Take another 10 breaths and still the mind.

LESSON THREE: PRACTISE MEDITATION

A Walking Meditation

1. *Walk slowly.*

2. *Focus on an image ahead.*

3. *Be aware of the sensations of breathing.*

4. *Pay attention to each inhalation and exhalation.*

5. *Count each inhalation up to 10 and then start all over again.*

6. *Rest and relax as a whole body breathing.*

7. *Open up to a growing peacefulness and love.*

8. *Feel the relaxation sinking into you, becoming a part of you.*

Lesson Four

Be Mindful

"We practice mindfulness by remembering to be present in all our waking moments."

—Jon Kabat-Zinn

Being mindful involves being where you are, slowing down and truly immersing every part of your being in the present moment.

Opportunities for mindfulness are available to us every day from eating, walking, cooking and cleaning, to spending time with family and friends.

Engaging fully with every one of our senses, with these things we do regularly, is a powerful way to strengthen our mind, body and spirit.

Life is so very short. Rushing through it robs yourself of truly experiencing it. Whilst your mind is in a trance, busy ruminating about the past or the future, you are asleep to whatever you are currently doing, taking your life for granted and missing special moments and experiences.

Whilst writing this, an acquaintance died very suddenly. He was 41 with two young children. He had no idea when he woke up on that warm July morning that this day was to be his last.

I wonder if he savoured that day. I wonder if he told

his family that he loved them. I wonder if he lived that day to the fullest.

Every day, I ask myself, *"What would I do if today was my last day?"*

With this in mind, I spend 5 minutes thinking about how I would treat my family and those others around me. I think about the things I would do, the people I would spend time with, and the moments I would be grateful for.

I find that this exercise improves my mood, highlighting how lucky I am and how much I have to be grateful for.

In the same way, I ask my hypnotherapy clients to slow down and to live each day as if it were their last. I ask them to focus on all the meaningful things they experience each day and to savour each moment by taking at least ten breaths during each one. At the same time, I ask them to notice any positive thoughts and any reasons as to why each particular experience is special or important to them. I also ask them to notice any sensations in their body and any other reactions they have, such as a smile or tears.

Overall, I ask my clients to be mindful each day.

There are so many daily practices during which you can be mindful, from mindful eating, during which you really live the experience – savouring the smells, textures and tastes of every morsel of food – to wearing an elastic band on your wrist and snapping it every half an hour to remind yourself to pay attention to the here and now.

But at the very core of every mindfulness exercise is The Observer.

The Observer is the non-judgmental awareness that exists independently of our thoughts and feelings.

Paying attention to the Observer allows us an element of detachment from day-to-day events, giving us the ability to recognise that we are not our thoughts, feelings or actions.

The following exercise will increase your understanding of the Observer.

It will enable you to notice your breathing, emotions and thoughts without reacting to them, almost as if

Lesson Four: Be Mindful

you are watching your reactions from another person's perspective. Watching from this neutral standpoint is a vital step in increasing your overall level of mindfulness.

This exercise will also increase your self-awareness, enabling you to slow down and change your thoughts, behaviour and emotional reactions to ones which will benefit you and enable you to be happier and to achieve your goals.

The Observer Exercise

1. *Take a deep breath.*
2. *Inhale energy.*
3. *Exhale tension and discomfort.*
4. *Tune into your body.*
5. *Invite your body to relax.*
6. *Notice any physical sensations.*

7. *Notice the weight of your body, the sensation of clothes on your skin, any warm or cool areas, any tension or discomfort and any relaxed areas of the body.*

8. *Think about the fact that you have all these sensations in your body, but you are not your body.*

9. *Notice that you are an observer of your sensations.*

10. *Notice any feelings or emotions.*

11. *Notice where you feel them in your body and what they feel like.*

12. *Think about the fact that you have feelings and emotions, but that you are not your feelings and emotions.*

13. *Notice that you are simply an observer of your feelings and emotions.*

14. *Watch your thoughts.*

15. *Notice any happy, sad or judgmental thoughts.*

Lesson Four: Be Mindful

16. Notice that you are not your thoughts and are simply an observer of them.

17. Take a deep breath and become aware of your body as a whole.

18. Take another 10 deep breaths and then let go and relax.

Lesson Five

Cultivate Self-Love

"Love is about becoming the right person. Don't look for the person you want to spend the rest of your life with; become the person you want to spend the rest of your life with."

—Neil Strauss

When I was a child, to accuse someone of loving themselves was the ultimate insult.

Those who loved themselves were deemed to be grandiose, narcissistic, arrogant and selfish. Being self-deprecating and actually disliking yourself was much more attractive at the time.

Famous comedians, Woody Allen and Joan Rivers (amongst others) gained popularity and notoriety for being underdogs who proudly displayed their insecurities and laughed at their many imperfections.

They both also wore self-hatred like a badge of honour.

Amongst so many self-directed insults, Woody Allen once famously stated: *"My one regret in life is that I am not someone else"* and Joan Rivers actually entitled one of her books: ***I Hate Everyone… Starting With Me.***

The truth of the matter, however, is that grandiosity, narcissism, arrogance and selfishness are actu-

Lesson Five: Cultivate Self-Love

ally traits of those lacking self-love; Jim Jones, Ted Bundy and Stalin being prime examples.

Rather, by fostering a loving relationship with ourselves, we increase our ability to be more empathetic and loving towards others.

The concept of loving and caring about ourselves above all others brings to mind every aeroplane emergency briefing, during which the steward or stewardess instructs us to think of ourselves first in case of an emergency.

I recall the last time I heard the instruction being when my youngest was only four. Although I had heard the instruction many times previously, for the first time, it actually struck a chord, making me question whether I could put myself first in such a potentially life and death situation.

Heart-wrenching as it would be, of course, it is the only logical thing to do in such an instance, since should we run out of oxygen, we would be rendered useless to help others in any event.

In the same way, in our day-to-day lives, once we start putting our needs and desires first, we can grow and develop as healthy and joyful human beings, after which we can look to help others.

Putting ourselves first includes viewing ourselves and treating ourselves in the best way possible, with the same care that we would treat our best friend, using a gentle tone of voice and supportive words.

We often take the miracle of our bodies and minds for granted, not realising that we are not infallible. We often hold ourselves up to an unachievably high standard and, unless we reach this standard, we berate ourselves as if we were an enemy.

When I was a teenager, I used to chant the words *"I hate myself"* over and over. I felt so uncomfortable in my own skin and I would continually feel embarrassed by my actions and reactions.

I often fantasised about being someone else, someone more beautiful, more outgoing and more popular. Even though my family and friends would try and build me up, nothing I did was ever good enough for me. I remember continually scolding myself.

LESSON FIVE: CULTIVATE SELF-LOVE

I stopped short of causing myself physical harm; however, some of my teenage clients do not. They wound themselves mentally and physically, which leads to even lower self-confidence and a knock to their physical well-being.

Over the years, I have taught myself to see the positives in my appearance and behaviour. I have learned how to accept and appreciate who I am.

The following exercises are geared towards teaching self-love, an essential part of our journey towards serenity, inner calm and finding happiness.

> ## *Loving Kindness Meditation*
>
> 1. *Inhale slowly. Allow your breath to flow through your body, from your head to your toes.*
> 2. *As you exhale, imagine all your concerns being washed away.*
> 3. *Think of someone who cares about you.*

4. *Picture them in front of you. Visualise their warmth, kindness and compassion.*

5. *Wish them well: "May you be safe, happy and healthy."*

6. *Imagine them returning the same good wishes to you: "May you be safe, happy and healthy."*

7. *Feel their warmth flowing towards you.*

8. *See yourself through their eyes with warmth, kindness and compassion.*

9. *Wish yourself well: "May I be safe, happy and healthy."*

10. *Think of your family and those closest to you.*

11. *Picture them in front of you. Feel their love and warmth.*

12. *Wish them well: "May you be safe, happy and healthy."*

13. *Think of your friends.*

LESSON FIVE: CULTIVATE SELF-LOVE

14. Picture them before you.

15. Wish them well: "May you be safe, happy and healthy".

16. Think of your neighbours, co-workers and other acquaintances.

17. Wish them well: "May you be safe, happy and healthy."

18. Imagine those with whom you have a difficult relationship or a misunderstanding.

19. Wish them well: "May you be safe, happy and healthy."

20. Extend goodwill to those who you don't know.

21. Wish goodwill to all the people in the world: "May you be safe, happy and healthy."

22. Extend goodwill to all life on our planet and beyond: "May you be safe, happy and healthy."

A 5-Minute Exercise to Induce Self-Love

1. *Put on some soft, instrumental music.*
2. *Close your eyes and smile.*
3. *Visualise a radiant light beaming down on you from above.*
4. *As you inhale, send love to yourself.*
5. *Feel the love flowing throughout your body.*
6. *As you exhale to the count of 5, imagine sending love to others.*
7. *Repeat the exercise for 5 minutes.*

LESSON FIVE: CULTIVATE SELF-LOVE

A 5-Minute Meditation on Self-Acceptance

1. *Stand in front of a full-length mirror.*

2. *Put yourself in the shoes of someone who cares about you.*

3. *Look into your eyes from this other person's perspective.*

4. *Look at each part of your body from your head to your toes.*

5. *Notice areas of beauty and accept every part of your body completely.*

6. *Spend 5 minutes repeating the words "I accept myself exactly as I am".*

Exercise to Increase Self-Compassion

1. *Think of times when you have been cared about by people or pets.*

2. *Imagine their loving feelings for you sinking into your body.*

3. *Think of people you have compassion for.*

4. *Get a sense of their worries and feel concern for them.*

5. *Put a hand on your chest and wish them well.*

6. *Let compassion fill you and flow through you.*

7. *Apply compassion to yourself.*

8. *Put a hand on your chest and wish yourself well.*

9. *Imagine compassion spreading throughout your entire body, soothing the hurt inside.*

Lesson Five: Cultivate Self-Love

Healing Your Inner Child

The idea that we all have an inner child was first suggested by psychologist Carl Jung and more recently, in 2010, by author, Caroline Myss, who suggested that an inner child is present within all of us.

According to Caroline Myss, the inner child "*establishes our perceptions of life, safety, nurture, loyalty, and family. Its many aspects include the Wounded Child, Abandoned or Orphan Child, Dependent, Innocent, Nature, and Divine Child.*"[6]

Overall, I have included the following exercise on healing your inner child for those readers who have unresolved issues relating to childhood.

By spending time on this exercise and healing your inner child, you will notice an increase in self-love.

---

6 https://web.archive.org/web/20120529044642/http://myss.com/library/contracts/four_archs.asp

Exercise to Heal Your Inner Child

1. Tune into your breathing.

2. Imagine your five-year-old self.

3. See your five-year-old self standing in front of you.

4. Kneel down in front of them, hold their hands and thank them for everything that they have done to help you.

5. Thank them for trying to please people to feel loved and accepted.

6. Tell them, "You are loved exactly as you are".

7. Tell them that they are loved because they are you.

8. Tell them, "There is nothing you have to say or do to be loved".

9. Give the child a hug and tell them that you love them.

10. Take a deep breath and say, "I am loved exactly as I am";

LESSON FIVE: CULTIVATE SELF-LOVE

> *"There is nothing I have to say or do to be loved".*
> *"I am simply loved for being me".*
>
> *11. Smile as you feel love flowing throughout your entire body.*

Lesson Six

Be More Confident

"Nothing can be done without hope and confidence."

—Helen Keller

Helen Keller utilised hope and confidence to reach success.

Helen was blind, deaf and unable to talk, and yet, in 1904, she graduated from college, creating history as the first blind and deaf person to do so.

She then went on to become an inspirational icon for the blind and deaf, a lecturer, a political activist and an author of twelve books.

The word *confidence* comes from the Latin word *fidere* meaning *to trust*.

Hence *self-confidence* literally means *self-trust*, a belief in your own ability to achieve your goals.

In an interview in 2017, Microsoft co-founder, Bill Gates, stated that he believed his self-confidence was key to his success.

In the interview, he stated that confidence was a vital personality trait, responsible for increasing a person's courage to overcome obstacles, as well as enabling them to find their passion.[7]

---

[7] https://www.cnbc.com/2017/10/24/why-bill-gates-says-you-need-confidence-to-achieve-success.html

Lesson Six: Be More Confident

The more self-confident a person is, the greater trust they have in their abilities. This leads to more passion, determination and motivation to take risks, which, in turn, leads to greater opportunities.

Self-confident people tend to reframe rejection and failure as learning opportunities. They deal with pressure and tackle personal and work-related challenges in a focused way, thus increasing both their inner strength and their ability to achieve their goals.

On the flip side, a lack of confidence will have a negative effect on moods, social interactions, achievements and career advancement.

When I was 24, I decided to pursue a Law Degree. I had just finished training as a teacher but felt dissatisfied and restless. Law had always been something that interested me.

I remember watching *L.A. Law* as a child in the 80s, after which I would daydream of silencing the courtroom with my own words of wisdom, feeling a surge of achievement when the criminals were thrown into jail by an imaginary Panel of Jurors.

My mum and dad, who always encouraged me to challenge myself, emotionally and financially supported the decision. It was a big decision for me. I doubted my ability to pass the course as well as my ability to find a job afterwards (Law was so heavily oversubscribed at the time). However, I pushed away my doubts and I applied and was then accepted at the College of Law in London.

I went on to complete the Law Conversion Degree followed with The Legal Practice Course, after which I found a job in the West End, in the area of Litigation, a role which mostly involved working behind a desk and drafting letters.

During the 5 years I spent hidden away in that office, I realised that being a solicitor in the UK had very little in common with the glamorous and exciting legal world portrayed in *L.A. Law*.

From my point of view, the job was completely devoid of all excitement which was further compounded by a feeling of hopelessness and boredom.

I felt powerless and controlled in every way.

Lesson Six: Be More Confident

I was bound by volumes and volumes of antiquated rules and regulations, and, at the same time, unable to exercise any autonomy or initiative, my every move being constantly monitored by my boss.

As time wore on, my relationship with him slowly disintegrated. He was looking to work with an assistant who idolised and blindly obeyed him, whereas I was the opposite. I was ambitious, passionate and enthusiastic, looking to be successful in my own right.

Ultimately, to cut a long story short, I lost it – both my temper and, eventually, my job.

And, at the same time, my biggest fear was realised. I had failed.

That being said, my brief brush with the law changed me.

Once I had recovered from the frustration of having failed, I looked back upon those 7 years of studying and then working as a solicitor with a new-found self-confidence.

I realised that I was capable of more than I had ever thought possible. I realised that I had the capability to achieve whatever goal I set myself.

Be confident in the knowledge that you have the ability to do the same. We are all capable of so much more than we can imagine.

Our brains and bodies are miraculous, designed to continually evolve and advance.[8]

By adopting a confident mindset, a deep trust in ourselves, we all have the ability to achieve our goals.

Increase your level of confidence with the following tips and techniques:

---

[8] https://www.ncbi.nlm.nih.gov/pmc/articles/PMC5649212/

Lesson Six: Be More Confident

1. Accept Everything About Yourself

A Meditation on Self-Acceptance

1. *Close your eyes and take a deep breath.*

2. *Notice any emotions (i.e. happiness, sadness, fear...). Accept them.*

3. *Be aware of each of your thoughts. Accept each thought.*

4. *Notice your breathing. Accept the sensations.*

5. *Notice any judgements. Accept them.*

6. *Notice any physical pain. Accept it.*

7. *Be aware of the different parts of your body.*

8. *Notice any sensations within each part. Accept them.*

9. *Embrace and accept yourself fully.*

2. Act As If You are Confident

The idea of *fake it till you make it* came from the theory of the self-fulfilling prophecy.

This theory states that if you are told something enough times, you start to internalise that message, turning it into a belief that eventually comes true.

An example of this can be seen by looking at method actors.

An actor preparing for a role actually becomes the new person. They do this by mimicking the other person's mannerisms, the way they walk and move, the way they talk and interact with others and by the things they tell themselves.

There are a number of studies showing that actors actually find it difficult to become themselves again.[9]

Use the following tips to help you act as if you are confident:

---

[9] https://royalsocietypublishing.org/doi/full/10.1098/rsos.181908

Lesson Six: Be More Confident

1. *Think positive thoughts such as: "I am attractive", "Someone cares about me".*

2. *Stand straight, with your shoulders back and with a genuine smile on your face.*

3. *Take up as much space as possible. Imagine doubling in size.*

4. *Relax your shoulders and hold your head up high when you walk.*

5. *Walk as if you have somewhere important to go.*

6. *When you enter a room, pause at the door and imagine a lovely smell that you want to inhale deeply.*

7. *When socialising, keep your voice low and gentle. Speak from the place you laugh from.*

3. Create an Anchor

An anchor is an association to a life memory. It is composed using one or any number of our senses, such as sight, sound, smell, taste or touch. Once created, the anchor can be used to recreate memories of times when we have felt at our best.

> ### *How to Create an Anchor*
>
> *1. Choose a positive state i.e. extreme confidence.*
>
> *2. Close your eyes and think of a time when you were extremely confident and at your best. Recreate the scene.*
>
> *3. Slow down your breathing*
>
> *4. Straighten your posture.*
>
> *5. Make the scene more colourful and louder.*
>
> *6. Make the picture bigger and brighter. Move it closer.*

LESSON SIX: BE MORE CONFIDENT

> 7. *Imagine the confident feelings in the pit of your stomach and then put your palm over it.*
>
> 8. *Infuse your favourite colour into the scene.*
>
> 9. *Set Your Anchor: Smell something powerful such as a lemon whilst your hands are in fists. Feel your nails dig in your hands and say "yes" into the pit of your stomach.*
>
> 10. *Repeat this twice.*

4. Boost Your Charisma

Charisma is the quality of being able to attract, charm and influence those around you. Charisma inspires confidence in others. It is one of the most essential traits of a successful person.

How to Increase Your Charisma When in a Social Situation

1. *Practise actively listening.*
2. *Take a genuine interest in the other person and focus on showing people that you like them.*
3. *Ask questions and listen more than you talk.*
4. *Whilst someone is speaking, continually bring yourself to the present moment by focusing on your breath and then put all your focus on the other person.*
5. *Hold eye contact with the other person for 3 seconds.*
6. *Whilst listening, keep your head still (imagine a book on your head).*
7. *Don't fidget.*
8. *Pause for 2 seconds before you speak.*
9. *Talk low and slowly.*
10. *Smile and use open body language.*
11. *Be comfortable and take up as much space as possible.*

5. Act Authentically

Being authentic is behaving in a way that exhibits how you really feel rather than showing people only a particular side of yourself. It is achieved by behaving as your true self, with courage and sincerity, regardless of your insecurities and imperfections.

An Exercise in Establishing Your True Self

1. *Recall a time when you were uncompromisingly you, passionate and in the moment.*

2. *How old were you?*

3. *Where were you?*

4. *What were you wearing?*

5. *Feel the emotions.*

6. *Think of adjectives to describe yourself during this experience, i.e. confident, glowing, graceful, happy, beautiful.*

7. *Watch yourself in a movie with those character traits.*

8. *What is your posture like?*

9. *How are you moving?*

10. *How are you speaking?*

11. *How are you interacting with other people?*

12. *Look in your eyes.*

13. *What are you thinking? How do you feel? What do you want?*

14. *Merge with your perfect you. Move as yourself.*

15. *Feel your power and beauty.*

16. *Before opening your eyes, hold your hands together as if in prayer.*

17. *Breathe slowly. Hold the position for 20-30 seconds.*

Lesson Seven

Pursue Your Dreams

"If you can dream it, you can do it."

—Walt Disney

Dreams provide us with a positive direction in life.

They give us a focus to move towards, motivating us to work harder and instilling excitement as we move closer and closer towards living our dreams.

As we work towards realising our dreams, goals are imperative, acting as clear signposts along the way.

Choosing ambitious but achievable goals gives our lives direction and brings a sense of accomplishment and satisfaction when we achieve them.

Ever since I attended a Tony Robbins 3-day event in 2007, a Seminar entitled *Unleash The Power Within*, during which I massaged the shoulders of a multitude of strangers, danced awkwardly to 2 Unlimited's *Tribal Dance* and walked barefoot over hot coals, I knew I wanted to work with other people to help them to achieve their goals.

Although I didn't achieve this dream straight away, it remained in my mind and, around ten years later, after remarrying, becoming a step-mum to two gorgeous girls, giving birth to another two beauti-

LESSON SEVEN: PURSUE YOUR DREAMS

ful babies and adopting three dogs, I commenced my hypnotherapy course.

I now work with clients daily, helping them achieve their goals at the same time as achieving mine.

Steps to Achieving Your Goals:

1. Have a Clear Goal in Mind

> ### *A Meditation on Goal Setting*
>
> *1. Say what you want 3 times.*
>
> *2. Take 5 deep breaths.*
>
> *3. Feel the sensation of relaxation passing through your body, from your head to your toes.*
>
> *4. Visualise a beautiful beach with light yellow sand and a clear blue sea*

5. Imagine sitting on the beach with your eyes closed. Hear the waves coming in and out. Feel the sand under your feet. Smell the sea.

6. Imagine walking in a garden. Smell the freshly cut grass and feel the wet dew under your feet.

7. Imagine feeling very cold and shivering.

8. Imagine feeling hot and sweating.

9. Grow to the size of a giant.

10. Shrink to the size of a freckle.

11. Imagine lying on the bed. Feel the bed against your body. Feel your body becoming heavier and heavier. Imagine all your tension melting into the bed.

12. Feel your body becoming lighter, more relaxed and weightless.

13. Repeat what you want 3 times. Imagine yourself achieving your goal.

2. Put Your Goal in Writing and Tell Someone Your Goal

A Meditation to Ask for Guidance in Achieving Your Goal

1. *Breathe in relaxation and breathe out tension 5 x.*

2. *Make sure that your exhalations are longer than your inhalations.*

3. *Invite each part of your body to soften and relax.*

4. *Visualise being in a peaceful place.*

5. *Notice the colours and shapes.*

6. *Notice the sounds, smells and temperature.*

7. *Tune in to your inner self.*

8. *Ask your inner wisdom specific questions and advice in relation to reaching your dream.*

9. *When you have understood the guidance, thank yourself.*

3. Address Any Worries or Obstacles Obstructing Your Goal.

An Exercise to Stamp Out Worries Blocking Your Goal

1. *Breathe in fresh air and energy, and breathe out tension.*
2. *Relax each part of your body.*
3. *Visualise being in a peaceful place.*
4. *Explore it.*
5. *See the sights, sounds and smells.*
6. *What time of day is it?*
7. *What is the temperature?*
8. *How are you dressed?*
9. *Visualise the outcome that you would like to see from the worry.*
10. *Imagine the best outcome.*
11. *Energise this image.*

LESSON SEVEN: PURSUE YOUR DREAMS

> *12. Let a word or phrase come to mind that represents this outcome.*
>
> *13. Any time in the future that you worry about this thing, take a deep breath and relax.*
>
> *14. Imagine a big red stop sign and stop the worrying thought.*
>
> *15. Become aware of the outcome that you desire and the phrase that reminds you of it.*
>
> *16. Imagine the outcome you desire coming true.*

4. Create a Written Plan On How to Execute Each Goal

> ### The Plan
>
> *1. Write down your goal.*
>
> *2. Take a sheet of paper and set a timer for 10 minutes and write down as many ideas as you can to reach this goal.*

3. *Delete unsuitable options and circle the most sensible ones.*

4. *Write a step-by-step action plan to accomplish the goal.*

Visualisation on Executing Your Goal

1. *Visualise being in a peaceful place.*

2. *What do you see, hear and smell?*

3. *Imagine resting in a comfortable place there.*

4. *Imagine carrying out your plan.*

5. *Imagine overcoming obstacles.*

6. *When you have completed the plan, notice where in your body you feel positive sensations.*

7. *Invite the feelings to grow larger and stronger.*

8. *Imagine the feelings spreading over your entire body.*

9. *Imagine carrying out the plan successfully again.*

10. *Do this 3 x.*

11. *Keep moving towards your goal.*

5. Trust That You Will Achieve Your Goal

Meditation for Achieving Your Goal

1. *Put your attention on your thoughts.*

2. *Repeat "I can achieve my goal".*

3. *Pay attention to the centre of your chest. Breathe in confidence.*

4. *Send confidence to your inner self.*

5. *Allow confidence to flow between your heart and your head.*

6. *Focus on what you want.*

7. *Imagine achieving your goal.*

8. *Visualise your goal as a golden light.*

9. *Then say "thank you" and know that you have received what you have asked for.*

Lesson Eight

Be Kind

"Be kind, don't judge and have respect for others. If we can all do this, the world would be a better place. The point is to teach this to the next generation."

—Jasmine Guinness

Being kind, having friendships and working effectively with others is a huge determinant of our level of happiness.

Research links kindness to a wealth of physical and emotional benefits.[10] Studies show that, amongst other benefits, kindness leads to an increase in happiness.[11]

My 73-year-old mother is a testament to this.

Not only is she the kindest person that I know, but she is also the happiest when she is helping others.

As a child, I remember the years she spent volunteering in the local Hospice, where she made so many friends and from where we seemed to acquire a constant stream of dinner guests.

If anyone needed a favour, my mother was the one to call.

---

10 https://pubmed.ncbi.nlm.nih.gov/29702043/
11 https://www.researchgate.net/publication/323927175_Happy_to_help_A_systematic_review_and_meta-analysis_of_the_effects_of_performing_acts_of_kindness_on_the_well-being_of_the_actor

Lesson Eight: Be Kind

Nothing was (and still is) ever too much for her.

Helping others actually fulfils an innate need within us.

This need can be seen when looking at our primate ancestors who foraged in groups to ensure their survival[12] and created a basic language, which, according to a recent study, may have evolved due to a need for advanced communication to share ideas. According to this study, this communication helped our ancestors to develop tools, enabling them to improve their lives and to evolve further.[13]

Hence social interactions and friendships have always been imperative to our evolution and survival.

Friendships actually have the ability to cure pain. There are a number of studies which conclude that the touch of a romantic partner can alleviate physical pain.[14]

Other studies have shown that those undergoing

---

12 https://www.nature.com/articles/nature10601
13 https://www.nature.com/articles/ncomms7029
14 https://www.ncbi.nlm.nih.gov/pmc/articles/PMC5468314/

chemotherapy for cancer tend to fare better if they have social support and social interactions.[15]

Overall, having friends and sharing rapport with others infuses a sense of security in us and ultimately leads to greater life satisfaction, peace and happiness.

Tips to Create Rapport with Others

1. *When you are introduced to someone, use a handshake that matches the strength of the other person.*

2. *Treat everyone you meet as if they are an old friend. Make sure that whoever you spend time with leaves feeling happier.*

3. *Alternatively, imagine that the person you are speaking with is the main part in a film you are watching.*

---

15 https://www.cambridge.org/core/journals/network-science/article/social-influence-on-5year-survival-in-a-longitudinal-chemotherapy-ward-copresence-network/4E08D5F5A0D332AA5BB119310833A244

Lesson Eight: Be Kind

4. *Really take the time to get to know other people, including those who you don't like. In the words of Abraham Lincoln "I don't like that man; I must get to know him better".*

5. *Don't take anything personally. Nothing other people do is because of you; it is because of themselves. Their words and actions are a result of their own memories, thoughts and beliefs.*

6. *Be more interested than interesting. People are interested in people interested in them.*

7. *After someone speaks, listen. Then let your facial expression react, pause for 2 seconds and then answer.*

8. *Rest the tip of your tongue at the base of your mouth when someone is talking so that you are not tempted to speak.*

9. *Repeat back what the other person said.*

10. *Look at people with a soft focus.*

11. *Smile or imagine smiling as you speak.*

> *12. Celebrate other people's accomplishments.*
>
> *13. Give genuine compliments and sincere praise to help others like themselves better.*

The Importance of Empathy

Kindness is an essential part of human nature and having empathy teaches us to be kinder to others. Empathy involves tuning in to the emotions of other people, tuning in to what they are experiencing and to what they need.

Learn to become more empathetic by following the steps below.

> *1. Cultivate an Empathetic Attitude:*
>
> *1.1. Listen to other people's point of view.*
> *1.2. Act as if you care and really want to understand the other person's pain.*
> *1.3. Mirror back what they say.*

Lesson Eight: Be Kind

> *1.4. Give everyone the benefit of the doubt as you do to yourself.*
>
> ## *2. Increase Your Emotional Empathy:*
>
> *2.1. Become attuned to other people's moods.*
> *2.2. Mirror other people's expressions and gestures.*
> *2.3. Discover other people's values.*
> *2.4. Learn about other people by listening to them discussing their relationships with their parents, partner and friends.*

Be Respectful to Others

Respect means showing someone that you accept them for who they are, even when they are different from you and even when you don't agree with them.

Respect in your relationships builds feelings of trust, safety, and well-being.

I read a quote from Albert Einstein earlier today which encapsulated the essence of respect perfectly:

"I speak to everyone in the same way, whether he is the garbage man or the president of the university."

Show respect to others as follows:

1. Use the acronym THINK before you speak.

- T – Is It True?
- H – Is It Helpful?
- I – Is It Inspiring?
- N – Is It Necessary?
- K – Is It Kind?

2. Accept Compliments Gracefully

2.1. After being given a compliment, pause.
2.2. Accept the compliment; enjoy it.
2.3. Let the acceptance show on your face.
2.4. Thank the person.

3. Thank People Properly

3.1. Thank the person for something specific they did.

3.2. Recognise the effort it took for the person to help.
"Thank you for making the effort to..."

3.3. Tell the person exactly what their help meant to you.

4. Apologise Properly

4.1. Acknowledge that you hurt the person and that you are truly sorry.

4.2. Listen to the other person vent.

4.3. Try not to become defensive.

4.4. Find some way to make amends.

4.5. Show them through your actions that you have learnt a lesson.

4.6. Do not make the same mistake again.

Lesson Nine

Learn to Deal with Negative Emotions

"The most important decision you make is to be in a good mood."

—Voltaire

Negativity is an obstacle to reaching your goals and living your best life.

It is natural to feel negative emotions, however, it is how you deal with them which can increase or decrease your quality of life and potential for later regrets.

As an extreme over-thinker, my thoughts have often been responsible for creating low moods.

In addition to this, I am incredibly sensitive to negativity in others, often blaming myself and taking things personally when they are not.

At times, this has been an obstacle to making a good first impression, building friendships and sustaining intimate relationships.

In the past, I have been described as "stand-offish" when, in reality, I am just cautious (afraid of being rejected and hurt) and so I really need to get used to situations and people before I jump in.

Over the years, I have worked hard to deal with,

LESSON NINE: LEARN TO DEAL WITH NEGATIVE EMOTIONS

what can only be described as, negative thoughts and emotions.

My early childhood strategy of pretending to be invisible whilst hiding behind mummy's skirt didn't seem to cut it as I grew older.

The tips below (which are based on Neuro-Linguistic Programming techniques) are ones that I use in my day-to-day life.

> *Dealing with Unhelpful Thoughts or Stories*
>
> 1. *Think of the negative thought or story.*
> 2. *Say, "I'm thinking about..."*
> 3. *Say to yourself, "I am in control of my thoughts. Why has this negative thought or story come up?"*
> 4. *Dispute the thought's validity. Say, "No, there are other ways of looking at this".*

5. *Stop judging or trying to find meaning in the thought or story. Negativity is exacerbated by our interpretations and judgements.*

6. *Only think about the things that are under your control, i.e. your thoughts and actions.*

7. *Ask yourself if the negativity is within your control. If it is not, let it go.*

8. *There is no point in over-analysing other people's reactions to you. Their reactions are a product of their own thoughts and are out of your control.*

9. *Take a third-person perspective. Watch the scenario on a TV screen.*

10. *Brainstorm ways to improve what's bothering you. Think about the ideas which will work and cross out those which won't.*

LESSON NINE: LEARN TO DEAL WITH NEGATIVE EMOTIONS

How to Deal with Negative Images

1. *Put negative images or video clips on an imaginary TV.*

2. *Turn the image upside down; turn down its colour and brightness.*

3. *Make the image smaller and smaller.*

4. *Move the image as far away from you as possible.*

5. *Destroy the image and replace it with a positive image instead.*

6. *Watch the new image. Make the new image brighter and brighter.*

7. *Move it closer and closer.*

8. *Step into your body in the new image. Notice what you are wearing, what you are doing and how others are responding to you.*

9. *Feel the positive feelings. Notice where they are in your body.*

10. *Listen to and note down your positive thoughts.*

Exercise to Replace Negativity with Positivity

1. *Think about the negativity. Feel the negativity.*

2. *Recall a time when you felt happy.*

3. *Intensify the happy experience.*

4. *Feel the happy experience in every part of your body.*

5. *Start visualising the negative and positive experiences at the same time.*

6. *Increase the positive feelings.*

7. *Feel the positivity soothing the negativity.*

8. *Feel the positivity comforting and reassuring the negativity.*

9. *Take 10 deep breaths as you connect to the positivity.*

Lesson Nine: Learn to Deal with Negative Emotions

Working with Anger

In my hypnotherapy sessions, anger is an emotion that many clients seek help with.

Uncontrolled anger can lead to both self-harming and harming others by using destructive words or with unrestrained negative physical behaviour.

Anger is simply panic. When we are angry, we are scared that other people's actions will leave us helpless, overwhelmed, betrayed and abandoned.

The issue with anger is that it causes a loss of control and completely detracts from any point we might want to make.

The following tips can help deal with anger:

The 10-10-10 Exercise

1. *Transport yourself to the future, to a time when you will be calm and unaffected.*

2. *Transport yourself 10 minutes from the current moment.*
   – Where will you be?
   – What will you be doing?
   – How do you feel about the situation now? Think about how much your anger will have reduced.

3. *Transport yourself 10 hours from the current moment.*
   – Where will you be?
   – What will you be doing?
   – How do you feel about the situation now? Think about how much your anger will have reduced.

4. *Transport yourself 10 days in the future.*
   – Where will you be?
   – What will you be doing?
   – How do you feel about the situation now? Think about how much your anger will have reduced.

Tips to Use When You Are Angry with Someone

1. *Think about the following questions for 3 days before reacting:*

    1.1. What have I received from that person?
    1.2. What have I given to that person?
    1.3. What problems have I caused that person?

2. *Try and remember that anger will exacerbate the situation so try and remain quiet while you allow the other person to explain themselves.*

3. *Try and understand their point of view and that behind their action is probably the need for attention.*

4. *Try to come to a compromise that suits all involved.*

> ### *A Meditation for Anger Management*
>
> 1. *Count slowly to 10.*
> 2. *Visualise a plastic shield around you where nothing can hurt you.*
> 3. *Press the thumb of one hand into the palm of the other hand.*
> 4. *Repeat "don't take it personally" 100 times.*

Dealing with Other People's Critiques

Anger is often sparked by criticism. Whilst being criticised, other emotions such as sadness, shame and even depression may also arise.

Throughout our life, we will be faced with other people's opinions and negative judgments and we will be unable to control them.

The following tips can help you deal with other people's criticisms:

Lesson Nine: Learn to Deal with Negative Emotions

> 1. *Accept and understand that if you create something and put it out there, it will stir up a response, positive or negative.*
>
> 2. *Listen to criticisms without feeling the need to defend yourself.*
>
> 3. *If the criticism is unfounded, remember that people are very slow to accept change and that they may be discouraging you simply because they are unused to seeing that side of you.*
>
> 4. *Remember that other people's criticisms are not within your control. Listen to them and then let them go.*

Lesson Ten

Learn to Deal with Other People's Negativity

"You cannot control the behaviour of others, but you can always choose how you respond to it."

—Roy T Bennett

To elaborate on the above quote, how you react to the behaviour of another can exacerbate or quash a situation.

Just today, I read a description of a friend's personality.

She had proudly posted the following on her Facebook feed: *"I have a heart of gold but my attitude is based on how you treat me"*.

In other words, *"I am a good person, but I will respond to you in a positive or negative manner depending on how I judge your treatment of me"*.

Lots of people would agree with the above (in fact, lots of people did with likes and love emojis).

Even going as far back as Leviticus 24, it says:

> *"And if a man cause a blemish in his neighbour; as he hath done, so shall it be done to him; Breach for breach, eye for eye, tooth for tooth: as he hath caused a blemish in a man, so shall it be done to him again."*

LESSON TEN: LEARN TO DEAL WITH OTHER PEOPLE'S NEGATIVITY

Times have not really changed in this regard, as responding in a like for like manner is still an acceptable reaction.

A former client, (who I shall call *John*) who suffered from low self-esteem and extreme mood swings, strongly believed in the maxim of spreading fire with fire.

If ever *John* felt aggrieved, rather than calmly attempting to resolve the situation, he would hurt the person in return, verbally or physically.

Sadly, rather than helping him in any way, this belief simply resulted in the eventual alienation of his family and friends.

Whilst working with *John* over several weeks, I attempted to show him the futility of this belief. I tried to highlight the fact that it provoked a circle of violence, rather than any calm resolution.

But, to no avail, *John* stubbornly held onto it and, as far as I am aware, he still lives alone, destroying one relationship after another.

In addition to the example above, when I typed in *an eye for an eye* on my Google search, the following two other real-life examples came up:

1. The murderer of Lee Rigby in 2013 (who was run over and then viciously stabbed to death due to his clothing and camouflage rucksack, signalling that he was in the armed forces) cited, repeatedly, that he had been motivated by his belief in the doctrine of an eye for an eye.

2. In 2017, an Iranian woman, wounded in an acid attack, was given the opportunity to have her attacker blinded with acid as per Sharia law.

In addition to these, there are numerous other historical and current examples to justify violence on the basis of an eye for an eye, from the atom bomb over Hiroshima in 1945 to avenge the attack on Pearl Harbour, to the continued usage of capital punishment in America.

As well as these, there are numerous other less extreme examples from cases of vigilante justice to petty playground bullying.

Lesson Ten: Learn to Deal with Other People's Negativity

I remain unconvinced of its validity, despite it being a widely accepted viewpoint.

Evidence shows that revenge is not actually so sweet.[16]

Responding in kind not only exacerbates the negativity but it also entrenches the negative behaviour as a neural pathway is formed leading to it being repeated.

Additionally, in the case of responding to verbal or physical violence in the same way, you are actually giving the behaviour that you don't like more power and credence, as well as not actually accepting responsibility for your own choices.

In my opinion, instead of reacting in kind, but by ignoring negative behaviour and refusing to get embroiled in the drama, in most cases you can stifle it.

The following techniques will help you to deal with most types of conflict in a controlled, rational and non-physically aggressive way.

---

16 https://www.psychologicalscience.org/observer/the-complicated-psychology-of-revenge

Tips for Dealing with Bullies and Other People's Negativity

1. *Don't take anything personally. Another person's negativity is not because of you. It is because of themselves. They may simply be trying to increase their own self-importance by putting you down. Alternatively, their negative behaviour may be a cover-up for their insecurities.*

2. *When someone is rude to you, before reacting, take 5 slow deep breaths and remove yourself from the situation, if possible.*

Tips for Dealing with an Angry Person

1. *Encourage the person to speak or rant.*

2. *Make eye contact.*

3. *Act politely. Say what you mean, but do not say it meanly.*

Lesson Ten: Learn to Deal with Other People's Negativity

4. *Start with a compliment and then concede something and find a point of agreement.*

5. *Get the message across to them that you think they are important, that their problem is important and that you are listening. Everyone wants to feel appreciated and understood.*

6. *Most importantly, don't argue, defend or make excuses.*

Tips for Improving Relationships and Dealing with Conflict

1. *Don't seek out unhealthy, spiteful gossip.*

2. *Find something to approve of in everyone. (Ironically, the traits we cannot tolerate in others are often the ones which we are unhappy with in ourselves).*

3. *Recognise everyone's positive traits and praise them.*

> 4. *Every time you talk about a conflict, recollect all the good things the person has done before citing anything negative.*
>
> 5. *Criticise privately and impersonally (solely criticising the behaviour).*
>
> 6. *When there is a conflict, remove yourself from the situation:*
>   – *Go for a walk.*
>   – *Write in a diary.*
>   – *Watch a film.*
>   – *Telephone a friend.*

Dealing with Passive Aggression and Silent Treatment

One of the most challenging types of negativity to deal with from others, comes in the form of passive aggression.

Passive aggression is a way of making your anger known, without physically or verbally communi-

Lesson Ten: Learn to Deal with Other People's Negativity

cating it directly. A few examples include rolling your eyes when someone is speaking, scowling and an overall refusal to engage in conversation, also known as The Silent Treatment.

In my family, I only ever encountered verbal aggression and it certainly was not passive.

When I behaved in a way that was unacceptable to those around me, an immediate verbal confrontation would ensue.

Passive aggression was not something I was familiar with until I met Bec.

We were both studying for our Legal Practice Course and became pretty close through our shared dislike of one of the Tutors.

Initially, it was pretty funny to laugh at the Tutor in question, however, the first red flag suddenly flew up, when she accidentally slammed the door in this Tutor's face.

Continuing on, the red flags began appearing all over the place.

From the way she used to tell me she would shun her boyfriend, when he upset her, to the fact that she would glare at people and mutter things about them under her breath.

And then one day she simply disappeared.

I continued to see her around the College but she simply ignored me completely. I never got to the bottom of exactly what I had done to offend her, but the pain caused by her silent treatment hurt me more than any other.

Several of my clients have also struggled to deal with passive aggression, often inflicted on them by their partners. Sometimes described as being in a Cold War, the pain inflicted is no less than overt acts of physical aggression.

The following tips can help you when faced with passive aggression or the silent treatment:

Lesson Ten: Learn to Deal with Other People's Negativity

1. *Acknowledge that this is the person's usual response to express anger or disapproval. They have chosen to be cold and controlling rather than having an actual conversation with you.*

2. *Know that you cannot control or change them, nor are you responsible for their behaviour. Hence, do not show any vulnerability as this gives them control so they can continue to manipulate the relationship to fit their style of communication.*

3. *Confront them a few days later, explaining the impact of the behaviour.*

In the meantime:

1. *Detach. Refuse to respond in any way to the behaviour in the hope that it will die away.*

2. *Observe the behaviour without any emotion at all, noting the following:*

    2.1. They may be looking for attention by acting the victim.
    2.2. They may be looking to avenge you.

> *2.3. They may be trying to show you that they cannot be controlled.*
>
> 3. *Overall, accept that they are not taking any responsibility for the problem.*
>
> 4. *With the above in mind, ignore the behaviour. Stop pushing, nagging or requesting. To their delight, you have been giving them attention. Now ask for nothing.*
>
> 5. *Refrain from having any interactions with them. Detach and do your own thing.*

Overcoming Negativity by Ignoring Unwanted Behaviour

As mentioned in the tips above, ignoring unwanted behaviour is often the best strategy.

In June 2006, Amy Sutherland wrote an essay in the New York Times, describing a wife's success in improving her husband's behaviour by using exotic-animal training techniques.

Lesson Ten: Learn to Deal with Other People's Negativity

The woman in question treated her husband in the same way as an animal trainer treats a misbehaving dolphin.

When the dolphin does something wrong, a trainer doesn't respond in any way. The trainer stands still, doesn't look at the dolphin and then returns to work.

The trainer ignores the unwanted behaviour.

In the same way as I mentioned earlier, any response, positive or negative, fuels another response. Whereas, if a behaviour provokes no response, if the behaviour is ignored, it dies away.

Confrontations

The above having been said, sometimes it is impossible not to respond to negative behaviour as confrontations are sometimes necessary in resolving disputes.

The following tips can be used when confronting someone about their behaviour:

1. *Begin by highlighting something positive that they have done and then explain gently why you are upset.*

2. *If they tell you that they don't want to discuss it, postpone the confrontation.*

3. *If they are willing to talk, ask them to explain why they are upset so that you can resolve things.*

4. *During the confrontation, be calm and present. Take deep breaths.*

5. *Look at both perspectives without any blame.*

6. *Realise that the underlying issue is that the other person is:*

    6.1. Needing to feel understood.
    6.2. Needing to be valued.
    6.3. Needing to be loved.

7. *Describe observations in a shared "we" phrase.*

8. *Find a solution that suits you both.*

Lesson Eleven

Practise Forgiveness

"I knew that I had to forgive in order to survive, in order to go on with my life without being overshadowed and possibly destroyed physically, mentally and emotionally by anger. I had to forgive".

—Scarlett Lewis

On 14th December 2012, Scarlett Lewis' 6-year-old son, Jesse, was murdered.

On that day, at Sandy Hook Elementary School, 20 children in total, between the ages of 6 and 7 years old, were shot and killed.

Despite her grief, Scarlett made a conscious decision to forgive her son's murderer.

As challenging as it can be, forgiving someone is incredibly important in order to release their power over you and to gain peace.

As the Buddha said, *"Holding onto anger is like drinking poison and expecting the other person to die."* Which is as ridiculous as it sounds.

Choosing to forgive someone who has hurt you doesn't mean that you excuse the behaviour, but by letting go of the anger, it frees you to focus on a more worthwhile cause.

Forgiveness really does have an inner power and a renewing effect. When we act with compassion and loving kindness towards ourselves and others, it allows us to let go of many negative feelings and emotions and is actually vital for both our mental and physical well-being.

> ## *Tips On Forgiving Another Person*
>
> *1. Think of someone who has hurt you.*
>
> *2. Imagine that person behaving in a hurtful or frustrating way.*
>
> *3. Put yourself in that person's shoes. Imagine what the person would say hurts or frustrates them about you.*
>
> *4. Imagine asking the person how much it upsets them to be upset with you.*
>
> *5. Imagine the other person describing something hurtful you did to them.*
>
> *6. Imagine apologising to each other.*

Meditation On Forgiving Others

1. *Visualise a compliment someone gave you.*

2. *Let the good feelings arise in your heart and infuse you with gratitude.*

3. *Open your heart and let love flow from it to everyone.*

    3.1. To family.
    3.2. To friends.
    3.3. To neighbours/strangers.
    3.4. To enemies.
    > *As the poet Henry Wadsworth Longfellow once wrote: "If we could read the secret history of our enemies, we should find in each man's life sorrow and suffering enough to disarm all hostility."*

    3.5. To the whole universe.

4. *Think of others as exactly the same as you. They all have a physical body and want to be happy.*

Lesson Eleven: Practise Forgiveness

> 5. *Put yourself in other people's positions. How would I feel? How would I want friends to treat me?*
>
> 6. *Imagine the person you need to forgive is someone that you love deeply.*

Lesson Twelve

Conquer Fear and Anxiety

"I experience anxiety from time to time. Here's a little trick that I use: Shake yourself free from fear and anxiety by inhaling deeply and hold your breath as you shake your left leg for a five-count; exhale and repeat with your right leg. Next, moving up your body, repeat with your hips, shoulders, arms, and wrists before finishing with your head and neck."

—Dr. Tasha Holland,
Licensed Mental Health Therapist

At Rickmansworth Hypnotherapy, I work with many clients suffering from anxiety.

Since Covid, these numbers have continued to increase and increase as so many people suffer from Covid's physical or mental after effects.

Whether related to Covid or not, each case of anxiety often follows a similar pattern.

It usually begins with a stimulus such as a negative thought or emotion.

This thought or emotion is perceived by the client to be dangerous or life threatening and hence, their body responds accordingly and prepares itself for the emergency.

Their breathing becomes more rapid, their heart begins to pound and their entire body becomes tense and ready for action. In extreme cases, the final result is often referred to as a panic attack whereby my clients have described becoming paralysed by fear, unable to breathe, shaky, dizzy, weak, numb or a combination of all of these.

Lesson Twelve : Conquer Fear and Anxiety

Also known as the fight or flight response, this likely developed from the survival needs of our early ancestors who would have required this emergency response to enable them to either fight or flee when faced with predators such as bears, sabre-toothed cats or giant birds.

Since much of the stress we experience in today's world is psychosocial stress, this ancient response which once was necessary for survival, can actually harm us, leading to a generalised panic disorder, suicidal thoughts and depression.

In my hypnotherapy sessions, I explain to my clients that deliberately relaxing is the cure for anxiety, since it is impossible to be completely relaxed and anxious at the same time.

I then go on to teach my clients techniques designed to relax them more deeply than ever, after which, I regress them to past times when they felt anxious. My aim is to change their habit of incorrect breathing and to rewire their brains so that they associate these past events with calm.

By learning to slow their breathing and to relax

more effectively, my clients manage to control their anxiety and eventually eliminate it altogether.

> ## *Tips on How to Respond to Anxiety*
>
> *1. Feel the sensations without getting upset or scared by them.*
>
> *2. Notice the thoughts that you are having.*
>
> *3. Treat them like clouds passing overhead. Label each one and let them float away.*
>
> *4. Shake the feeling out:*
>
> *4.1. Tap your feet.*
> *4.2. Bounce your knees.*
> *4.3. Shake your hands and legs.*
>
> *5. Stick your chest out.*
>
> *6. Put your head back.*
>
> *7. Put the biggest smile on your face.*
>
> *8. Breathe in as you slowly count to 5 in your mind, "1, 2, 3, 4, 5".*
>
> *9. Then breathe out as you count to 7.*

Lesson Twelve : Conquer Fear and Anxiety

10. *Imagine a bright light above your head. Allow the light to fill your body with a warm, relaxing feeling.*

11. *Cross your arms and put one hand on each shoulder.*

12. *Now move your hands down your arms to your fingers, and then back again.*

13. *Stroke your cheeks with the back of your hands.*

14. *Occupy yourself with an activity.*

An Exercise to Deal with Anxiety – the 333 Rule

1. *Name three sounds you can hear.*

2. *Name three things you see.*

3. *Move three parts of your body, for example, your fingers, legs and toes.*

More Tips for Dealing with Painful Feelings

1. *Think of a situation that induces anxiety.*

2. *Observe the feelings in your body.*

    2.1. Where are they?
    2.2. What shape are they?
    2.3. Are they light or heavy?
    2.4. Are they moving or still?
    2.5. Are they warm or cool?

3. *Breathe into the feelings taking slow, deep breaths.*

4. *As your breath flows in and around the feelings, imagine creating extra space in your body, so you are giving them room to move.*

5. *Allow the feelings to be there. Accept them.*

6. *Expand awareness to the present moment. What is happening right now? What can you see, hear or smell?*

7. *Reframe the feelings as excitement.*

LESSON TWELVE : CONQUER FEAR AND ANXIETY

Breathing for Anxiety and Pain Reduction

1. *Place one hand on your stomach and your other hand in the middle of your chest.*

2. *Take 20 deep breaths, fully breathing in and then breathing out slowly and letting go.*

3. *Try to make your breaths longer and slower.*

4. *As you breathe in, allow the breath to surround all the tension or pain in your body.*

5. *As you breathe out, imagine stress and tension leaving your body.*

6. *Continue breathing and focus your mind and breathing on relaxing areas of your body that are tense or painful.*

Lesson Thirteen

Embrace Failure

"I have not failed, I have found 10,000 ways that don't work."

—Thomas Edison

Despite his teachers saying that he was too *"stupid"* to learn, and his first two employers who fired him for being *"non-productive"*, Thomas Edison went on to invent both the lightbulb (after 1000 unsuccessful attempts) and a more efficient rechargeable battery (after 10,000 attempts).

As can be seen in the case of Thomas Edison, failure is not a step backwards. Rather, trial and error is often an excellent way to move out of our comfort zone, to overcome our fear of failure and to step closer towards success.

The most progressive companies deliberately seek employees with track records reflecting both failure and success, since an employee who has overcome failure will have gained both knowledge and experience and will have demonstrated an unwavering perseverance and courage in continuing with their goal.

Hence failure is very important for success and it is imperative to view each negative incident, each failure, as a learning experience and a way to improve oneself.

Lesson Thirteen: Embrace Failure

Exercise to Use When You F**K up

1. When you f**k up, pause for 5 seconds.
2. Acknowledge your feelings with words.
3. Then close your eyes for one minute and do not talk to anyone.
4. Breathe slowly with your eyes closed.
5. Keep breathing from 1-5 and say "Oh F**k" at the same time.
6. Find a solution. How can you make the best of the situation?
7. Open your eyes and do what you need to do.

How to Increase Your Emotional Resilience

1. Don't take things personally.
2. Look at the bigger picture and accept the fact that there are many factors involved.

> *3. Face your fears and acknowledge that every experience is a learning tool.*

How to Deal with Rejection

1. Make every "no" and every rejection empowering. Hearing "no" over and over and not quitting builds character.

2. When you stumble, try to pick yourself up and go about your way as if nothing had happened.

3. Do something every day that scares you.

4. Numb yourself to the word no. The word no means "not yet". When you get a no, ask why.

Lesson Thirteen: Embrace Failure

How to Deal with Failures

1. *Realise you are experiencing a setback.*
2. *Whether you feel angry, afraid, upset or any other negative emotion, know that your animalistic impulses are kicking in.*
3. *Imagine that this failure is a test for you.*
4. *Be rational. Know that you can handle this situation.*
5. *Do not give in to impulses. Instead, remind yourself of how strong and resilient you are.*

When You Fail

1. Write it down.

2. Write down the answers to the following:

   2.1. How can I do this better?

   2.2. Am I missing a crucial element that would make things easier or more efficient?

   2.3. What can I learn from this? How will I do it differently next time?

   2.4. What was the flaw? What needs to be fixed?

   2.5. What assumptions were wrong and need to be reevaluated?

3. Learn one thing from each failure.

Lesson Fourteen

Accept Death

"Do not fear death, but welcome it, since it too comes from nature. For just as we are young and grow old, and flourish and reach maturity, have teeth and a beard and grey hairs, conceive, become pregnant, and bring forth new life, and all the other natural processes that follow the seasons of our existence, so also do we have death. A thoughtful person will never take death lightly, impatiently, or scornfully, but will wait for it as one of life's natural processes."

—Marcus Aurelius

On 20th March 2020, my children's primary school, along with all the other schools, nurseries and colleges in the Country, closed. Globally, as a direct result of a pandemic, the scale of which had not been seen since the Spanish Flu of 1918, the world had gone into lockdown. I, alike so many others, had never witnessed anything like it.

My children, who I always had to drag out of bed in the mornings, who always seemed to feel sick, have a headache or pain in their legs just before we left the house to go to school, all of a sudden were bereft. My youngest, who was 5, was particularly affected. She would cry in the day, missing her friends and in her sleep, she would often call out *"Mummy, please don't die"*.

Just 8 days previously, Boris Johnson's infamous statement on 12th March 2020, had already brought home the severity of the upcoming situation, highlighting how close we all were to death.

His words *"I must level with you the British Public. Many more families are going to lose their loved ones*

Lesson Fourteen: Accept Death

before their time"[17] were received with shock and absolute terror.

With no better solutions, except for us all to flee the scene and isolate in our homes, death seemed to be inching closer by the minute.

And with the impending arrival of death for ourselves or our loved ones, for the first time in many of our lives, we were actually forced to think and talk openly about it.

There were some, of course, who ignored the topic, throwing themselves into whatever distraction they could find, from attempting to be the most enthusiastic homeschool teacher to becoming the most capable and creative household painters and decorators.

But whether addressed or ignored, the idea of death still conjured up painful emotions in the forefront or the background.

Human beings have always strived for survival, and death is the complete antithesis of this. Hence the

---

17 https://www.gov.uk/government/speeches/pm-statement-on-coronavirus-12-march-2020

reason we try to ignore it, rarely uttering the word for fear it could lead death directly to our front door.

Death is one of the few certainties that we have in life and so it is illogical to attempt to ignore it. Instead, we really need to accept that it will happen and prepare for it.

Knowing that each day that we live we are one day closer to our physical death and that our story is finite gives us a unique perspective and brings a richness to life. It allows us to savour each experience more deeply. It provides us with context on the preciousness of life and what really matters.

Some people act like they will live forever, always assuming that they have one more day. They get lost in the rat race and don't take the time to appreciate the relationships they have, the view of the sunset, the stars, a child's laughter…

When we realise that tomorrow may not exist for us, these tiny beautiful moments take on a much greater value. Time slows and we really appreciate every second.

Lesson Fourteen: Accept Death

In the words of Steve Jobs, two years after being diagnosed with Pancreatic Cancer: *"Remembering that I'll be dead soon is the most important tool I've ever encountered to help me make the big choices in life. Because almost everything – all external expectations, all pride, all fear of embarrassment or failure – these things just fall away in the face of death, leaving only what is truly important."*

What Is Death?

Death is a part of our day to day lives. Every moment is born and then it dies. Every cell, every neurone, every molecule, every being and every relationship will eventually come apart. Everything is transient, from the leaves on the trees, the seasons and the weather and even our thoughts come and go.

And life too is impermanent.

In dying, we lose everyone and everything that we have ever loved. We lose our dreams and our future. However, this loss of our lives relates solely to our physicality.

Fear subsides as we understand that we also have a non-physical presence.

This non-physical presence is eternal. It is the basic essence of who we are and it can never be changed. It can never get sick and can never die.

Become Comfortable with The Idea of Death

"When conditions are sufficient, a cloud transforms into rain, snow or hail. The cloud has never been born and it will never die. This insight of signlessness and interbeing helps us recognise that all lives continue in different forms. Nothing is created, nothing is destroyed, everything is in transformation."

—Thich Nhat Hanh

Upon death, our body simply ceases to exist in its current form.

Many spiritual traditions have suggested that all life is composed of the following 4 elements:

Lesson Fourteen: Accept Death

1. Earth;
2. Water;
3. Fire; and
4. Air.

They suggest that upon death, these 4 elements dissolve and return to nature in the ways described below:

1. The earth element, our physical form, stops moving and dissolves into water.
2. The water element dries up. Our bodies become incontinent, unable to ingest liquids and drain themselves of the water within. The water then dissolves into the fire element.
3. The fire element then causes the body temperature to rise and then fall.
4. After this, the body becomes cold and dissolves into air.
5. Finally, all that is left is breath; breath which is fast and then slow and then, eventually, disappears altogether.

A Meditation to Practise in Advance of Your Future Death

1. *Sit quietly.*

2. *Visualise a bright light.*

3. *Believe all the love and strength in the world is embodied within the light.*

4. *Merge with the light.*

5. *Imagine the light filling your body and mind.*

6. *Imagine it filling you with love and energy, strength and compassion.*

7. *Imagine it purifying, healing, empowering and enlightening you.*

8. *Imagine the light purifying negativity from your words.*

9. *Imagine the light cleansing all negativity from your feelings.*

10. *Rest in its warmth.*

LESSON FOURTEEN: ACCEPT DEATH

> *Meditation to Practise During Your Actual Death*
>
> 1. *Visualise a bright light.*
>
> 2. *Imagine the light cleansing all negativity from your body.*
>
> 3. *Imagine being healed by the light.*
>
> 4. *Imagine merging with the light.*
>
> 5. *Rest in its light and warmth.*

How to Help Those Who Are Dying

"Tell your friend that in his death, a part of you dies and goes with him. Wherever he goes, you also go. He will not be alone."

—JUDDU KRISHNAMURTI

Being supportive to someone who is dying is about letting go of our own fears, feelings of helplessness or our selfish needs to feel like we're doing something to make things better. Most of the time, the best we can do is just to be there with them, letting them know that we see what they're going through and that we care.

> *Exercise to Awaken Compassion for Those Who Are Dying*
>
> 1. *Imagine someone you care for in front of you.*
> 2. *Imagine their pain.*
> 3. *Feel your heart open and feel all of their suffering gathering into a mass of hot smoke.*
> 4. *As you breathe in, breathe in the smoke to your heart to purify all negativity and pain.*
> 5. *As you breathe out, send peace, happiness and healing to your friend.*

LESSON FOURTEEN: ACCEPT DEATH

Dealing with Grief

"Goodbyes are only for those who love with their eyes, because for those that love with their heart and mind there is no such thing as separation."

—RUMI

The following tips can help if you have just lost someone you love:

1. *Let yourself feel the pain and all the other emotions.*

2. *Be patient with the process. Accept that you need to experience your pain, your emotions, and your own way of healing, all in your own time.*

3. *Cry. Acknowledge all your feelings, including the ones you don't like.*

4. *Talk about your memories and the life of the person you lost.*

5. *Get support. Join a bereavement group.*

6. *Try to maintain your normal lifestyle and retain a sense of security. Ideally, don't change relationships, jobs or move home etc. during the first year of bereavement.*

7. *When you feel ready, do something creative:*

    7.1. Write a letter to the person who died, mentioning everything you wish you could say to them.
    7.2. Keep a journal.
    7.3. Make a scrapbook.
    7.4. Paint some pictures.
    7.5. Plant a tree.
    7.6. Involve yourself in a cause or activity in honour of the deceased.

Meditation If Suffering Grief

1. Visualise a bright light.

2. Open your heart and ask for help with your pain and suffering.

3. Visualise the light filling your heart and transforming your suffering into happiness.

4. Imagine happiness overflowing you. Imagine a stream of golden light flowing into your heart, transforming your suffering into joy.

5. Feel the warmth from the light healing you, soothing the pain.

6. Send the healing light to the one who died.

Releasing Regrets in Relation to the Deceased

1. *Grieve and say what is in your heart and mind to your loved one who has died.*

2. *Visualise the dead person looking at you with love and understanding.*

3. *Know that they want you to understand that they love you and forgive you and want to receive your forgiveness.*

4. *Allow your heart to open and put into words any hurt and then let go of that hurt completely.*

5. *Let forgiveness go to the dead person.*

6. *Tell them your regrets for any pain you caused.*

7. *Feel their forgiveness and love streaming towards you.*

8. *Know you are lovable and deserve to be forgiven and feel your grief dissolve.*

9. *Imagine them leaving, calm, happier and peaceful.*

Final Thoughts

"Perfection of character is this: to live each day as if it were your last, without frenzy, without apathy, without pretence."

—Marcus Aurelius

Live each day as if it were your last by practising the following:

> 1. *Express gratitude for everyone and everything in your life.*
>
> 2. *Cherish your family and friends. Tell them that you love them every single day.*
>
> 3. *Seek out things that make you happy. Change things that don't.*
>
> 4. *Give 100% to everything you do.*
>
> 5. *Listen carefully to other people's advice. Even if you do not agree or follow it, it will open you up to a different way of looking at things.*
>
> 6. *Increase your knowledge. Read as many books as you can and learn more about topics that interest you.*
>
> 7. *Seek out relationships with those who build you up and respect you. Ignore unwanted behaviour and those who treat you badly.*

> 8. *Remember, the way people treat you is a reflection of themselves. Hence, try not to harbour grudges.*
>
> 9. *And finally, as far as possible, let go of memories, thoughts and emotions that are hurtful to you.*

The following story is a very famous Buddhist parable about letting go:

> *"A senior and junior monk were walking down a path together and they arrived at a river with a strong current. As they prepared to cross the river, they saw a beautiful woman. She asked the monks for help to cross the river. The senior monk carried the woman on his shoulder and then set her gently down on the other side. They then parted ways.*
> *A bit later, the senior monk noticed that the junior monk was upset and asked him if something was bothering him.*

The junior monk explained that he was upset that the senior monk had carried the woman, since they were not permitted to touch women. The senior monk responded, "I left the woman hours ago at the bank, however, you still seem to be carrying her."

We spend so much time in our day-to-day lives worrying about what has happened or what might happen. Let go of all of that.

No matter how long you live, life is too short to focus on these things.

So savour each and every moment, smile, especially when you don't feel like it, and deliberately choose to be happy.

> *"Being happy doesn't mean that everything is perfect. It means that you've decided to look beyond the imperfections."*
>
> —Gerard Way